Cambridge Elements ≡

Elements of Improving Quality and Safety in Healthcare
edited by
Mary Dixon-Woods,[*] Katrina Brown,[*] Sonja Marjanovic,[†]
Tom Ling,[†] Ellen Perry,[*] and Graham Martin[*]
*THIS Institute (The Healthcare Improvement Studies Institute)
†RAND Europe*

MAKING CULTURE CHANGE HAPPEN

Russell Mannion

Health Services Management Centre, University of Birmingham

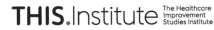

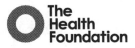

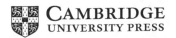

CAMBRIDGE
UNIVERSITY PRESS

University Printing House, Cambridge CB2 8BS, United Kingdom

One Liberty Plaza, 20th Floor, New York, NY 10006, USA

477 Williamstown Road, Port Melbourne, VIC 3207, Australia

314–321, 3rd Floor, Plot 3, Splendor Forum, Jasola District Centre,
New Delhi – 110025, India

103 Penang Road, #05–06/07, Visioncrest Commercial, Singapore 238467

Cambridge University Press is part of the University of Cambridge.

It furthers the University's mission by disseminating knowledge in the pursuit of
education, learning, and research at the highest international levels of excellence.

www.cambridge.org
Information on this title: www.cambridge.org/9781009236904
DOI: 10.1017/9781009236935

First published 2022

A catalogue record for this publication is available from the British Library.

ISBN 978-1-009-23690-4 Paperback
ISSN 2754-2912 (online)
ISSN 2754-2904 (print)

Cambridge University Press has no responsibility for the persistence or accuracy of URLs for
external or third-party internet websites referred to in this publication
and does not guarantee that any content on such websites is, or will remain,
accurate or appropriate.

Every effort has been made in preparing this Element to provide accurate and up-to-date
information that is in accord with accepted standards and practice at the time of publication. Although case histories are drawn from actual cases, every effort has been made to
disguise the identities of the individuals involved. Nevertheless, the authors, editors, and
publishers can make no warranties that the information contained herein is totally free from
error, not least because clinical standards are constantly changing through research and
regulation. The authors, editors, and publishers therefore disclaim all liability for direct or
consequential damages resulting from the use of material contained in this Element.
Readers are strongly advised to pay careful attention to information provided by the
manufacturer of any drugs or equipment that they plan to use.

Making Culture Change Happen

Elements of Improving Quality and Safety in Healthcare

DOI: 10.1017/9781009236935
First published online: October 2022

Russell Mannion
Health Services Management Centre, University of Birmingham

Author for correspondence: Russell Mannion, r.mannion@bham.ac.uk

Abstract: Healthcare policy frequently invokes notions of cultural change as a means of achieving improvement and good quality care. This Element unpacks what is meant by organisational culture and explores the evidence for linking culture to healthcare quality and performance. It considers the origins of interest in managing culture within healthcare, conceptual frameworks for understanding culture change, and approaches and tools for measuring the impact of culture on quality and performance. It considers potential facilitators of successful culture change and looks forward towards an emerging research agenda. As the evidence base to support culture change is rather thin, a more realistic assessment of the task of cultural transformation in healthcare is warranted. Simplistic attempts to manage or engineer culture change from above are unlikely to bear fruit; rather, efforts should be sensitive to the complexity and highly stratified nature of culture in an organisation as vast and diffuse as the National Health Service. This title is also available as Open Access on Cambridge Core.

Keywords: culture change, organisational culture, leadership, management, healthcare improvement

ISBNs: 9781009236904 (PB), 9781009236935 (OC)
ISSNs: 2754-2912 (online), 2754-2904 (print)

Contents

1 Introduction

The language of culture change has become commonplace in health reform. Cultural aspects of healthcare delivery are now widely regarded as important to quality of care, whether through fostering excellence or contributing to failure. Implicit in this thinking is the notion that there are good and bad cultures and that creating the right kind of culture will facilitate high-quality care. As a result, policy rhetoric frequently invokes the need to create and sustain a whole range of desirable cultures (e.g. open, compassionate, resilient, learning) and stamp out so-called toxic cultures (e.g. blame, fear, bullying, silence, club).

Yet culture is a slippery and elusive concept. It remains unclear whether talk of culture and culture change is largely empty flourish, or whether framing healthcare organisations in cultural terms offers useful insights and practical tools that might help to drive improvements. What do we actually mean when we talk of culture in health services? How are cultures linked to quality and safety? And can healthcare cultures be successfully moulded and harnessed to beneficial effect?

This Element addresses such questions. In doing so, it links conceptual and theoretical framings to empirical evidence and applications in practice. As a starting point, it traces the origins of the current interest in managing culture as a lever for health improvement (Section 2). The central sections of the Element unpack what is meant by organisational culture, introducing some of the principal frameworks and sources of ideas for understanding culture and culture change in healthcare contexts (Sections 3 and 4). The Element concludes by drawing together the key insights for those thinking about using cultural approaches to support improvement in healthcare organisations (Section 5). In general, the discussion is relevant to all staff working in healthcare settings, but where particular issues apply to specific professional groups, such as doctors or managers, this is noted.

2 The Origins of Current Interest in Organisational Culture

Interest in culture is not new. The origins of the term date back to Roman times: 'culture' is a derivation of the Latin *cultura* meaning to cultivate crops, in the sense of tilling the ground.[1] By the mid-modern era, its use had extended to the cultivation of individuals and attached to ideas of personal improvement – the cultivation of the self, for example, through education and through a refinement of social sensibilities in the realm of aesthetics, literature, and the arts. By the nineteenth century, social anthropologists studying indigenous peoples often used the metaphor of culture to explore the processes, rituals, and institutions (family, community, and religious) that supported the socialisation of individuals into shared practices. From here, it was a small step to seeing the study of organisations as akin to unravelling the cultural practices of indigenous peoples.

2.1 Developing the Concept of Organisational Culture

A number of US academic authors in the post-war period emphasised the importance of culture in shaping organisational behaviour and effectiveness.[2] Jaques, in his book *The Changing Culture of a Factory*, is credited with being the first scholar explicitly to refer to culture in an organisational context.[3] Two decades later, Pettigrew coined the term 'organisational culture' in his article, 'On studying organizational cultures'.[4] In the early 1980s, the concept entered mainstream management thinking through bestselling – if controversial – management handbooks written by US management gurus. Popularising the notion that corporate culture was a critical determinant of organisational performance, perhaps the most influential of these 1980s writings, outselling all other non-fiction books of the year, was Peters and Waterman's *In Search of Excellence: Lessons from America's Best-Run Companies*.[5] This book summarised research on the organisational attributes thought to distinguish 'excellent' companies from the less excellent (something that became problematic later on when many of the companies identified as paragons went out of business).

A key theme running through popular management books at the time was the apparent need for strong cultures, which were thought to be a critical factor in organisational success. Various strategies were put forward for how managers could manage and shape their company's culture. In their book *Corporate Cultures: The Rites and Rituals of Corporate Life*,[6] Deal and Kennedy examine hundreds of private companies in the USA. They claim to have identified four generic organisational cultures: the 'tough guy, macho culture', the 'work hard/ play hard culture', the 'bet your company culture', and the 'process culture'. Deal and Kennedy even make the bold (though unsubstantiated) assertion that the successful management of culture could yield an additional two hours of productive work per employee, per day.

Some of the early interest in organisational culture was fuelled, in part, by Japan's economic success and the perceived threat Japanese competitors seemed to pose to American businesses.[7] This sparked a keen desire to understand Japanese management practices and their cultural values.[8] It was hoped that by shaping an organisation's culture, it should be possible to transplant, for example, the cultural strengths of a Toyota or a Mitsubishi into a General Motors, creating cultural hybrids that Ouchi termed 'Z' companies.[9,10] The overall tenor and underlying structure of these popular management books, frequently rooted in the consultancy backgrounds of the authors, have been criticised for being more similar to the chatty and anecdotal style of business self-help texts than to academic writing.[11] Nevertheless, they were a runaway success and, in combination with journalistic outputs in the same vein, they sparked a widespread revolution in management thinking and practice. Although it was subsequently criticised extensively on methodological and practical grounds, this body of work was influential in drawing managerial attention to the informal aspects of organisational life and how these could be harnessed for improved performance.[12]

2.2 Managing Organisational Culture in Healthcare

Over the past two decades, interest in organisational culture within healthcare has grown apace. From the private sector's early fascination with the idea, the notion of organisational culture then moved on to captivate the healthcare sector, and a body of literature devoted to ideas and practical approaches to shaping and managing healthcare cultures has burgeoned. At the turn of the century, the publication of landmark reports highlighting the scale of harm to patients in the USA,[13,14] as well as in the UK,[15] identified organisational systems and cultures as key components of health system redesign. Ideas of culture subsequently became central to discussions of how to improve quality and safety, ranging from sustained improvement collaboratives to business process re-engineering and Lean production systems.[16] (For more information on these areas, see the Elements on audit, feedback, and behaviour change,[17] Lean and associated techniques for process improvement,[18] and collaboration-based approaches.[19])

A succession of high-profile inquiries into widespread failures in quality and safety in the National Health Service (NHS) subsequently alighted on organisational culture as the primary culprit at the root of scandals. In 2001, for instance, the public inquiry into failings in children's heart surgery at Bristol Royal Infirmary[20] concluded that the culture of healthcare in the NHS 'which so critically affects all other aspects of the service which patients receive, must develop and change'. The inquiry described the prevailing culture at the Bristol Royal Infirmary at the time of the tragic events as a 'club culture', which focused excessive power and influence around a core group of senior managers. The report pinpoints the cultural characteristics of an NHS that had colluded in fostering an environment where dysfunctional behaviour and malpractice were not effectively challenged, and it highlights a number of cultural shifts seen as necessary to transform the NHS into a high-quality, safety-focused institution, one that is sensitive and responsive to the needs of patients.

These same themes emerged again a decade later when the public inquiry report into Mid Staffordshire surfaced similar organisational failings, which were implicated in contributing to the deaths of hundreds of patients between 2005 and 2009. The report states that there was an 'insidious negative culture involving a tolerance of poor standards and a disengagement from managerial and leadership responsibilities'. It concludes that the 'extent of the failure of the system shown in this Inquiry's report suggests that a fundamental culture change is needed'.[21] Such concerns remain current: in 2018, a report into an NHS scandal – examining more than 450 premature deaths in the 1990s at Gosport War Memorial Hospital – invoked culture 21 times. The report included the suggestion that a 'culture of "doctor knows best" prevailed' and that this was a major cause of service failings in the hospital.[22]

Culture is periodically rediscovered and identified as both the culprit and solution to failings in patient care. Yet implementation of recommendations is often weak – in part because lack of recognition of the complexities of culture[23] is seemingly dooming the NHS to repeat the same mistakes.[24] In fact, cultural reform is so often prescribed in response to health service failures[20–22,25] that recommendations to change culture have something of a Groundhog Day quality.[26]

Box 1 provides details of an intervention case study at a US academic medical centre, which is designed to create a supportive culture for employees to voice concerns about unprofessional behaviour.

BOX 1 CREATING A CULTURE THAT SUPPORTS EMPLOYEES IN RAISING CONCERNS ABOUT TRANSGRESSIVE AND DISRUPTIVE BEHAVIOURS

Healthcare scandals in the NHS and elsewhere have highlighted the vital role of employees in raising concerns and speaking up about poor quality care, as well as the importance of organisations responding appropriately when such concerns are raised.

A 2019 intervention case study in a US academic medical centre (John Hopkins Medicine) aimed to explore the organisational barriers to employee voice and make improvements to organisational cultures and processes so that the organisation was better able to identify and respond to employee concerns in relation to addressing transgressive or disruptive behaviours.[27] The diagnostic interviews identified a 'culture of fear' pervading the organisation, with individuals holding positions of power colloquially known as 'untouchables' who engaged in transgressive or disruptive behaviour with apparent impunity. Widely held perceptions about the likely response to concerns discouraged staff from speaking up.

In response to the study findings, a structured intervention programme was implemented in the organisation to develop a more open culture and thereby encourage employee voice. This centred around four actions:

- sharing the interview findings
- coordinating and formalising mechanisms for identifying and dealing with disruptive behaviour
- training leaders in encouraging voice among employees
- building capacity to facilitate difficult conversations.

The authors conclude that the interventions appear to have had some impact on developing a more open culture; not least because of the benefits from removing several 'problematic' senior individuals from positions of power within the organisation.

3 What Is Organisational Culture?

We now turn to how organisational culture has been conceptualised in the literature. The following subsections explore rival interpretations of culture (Section 3.1) and how culture is layered (Section 3.2) and forms into subcultures in healthcare organisations (Section 3.3).

3.1 Conceptualising Organisational Culture

Definitions of organisational culture abound.[28–30] Some are colloquial and rather vague: 'the way things are done around here' (note that 'here' may comprise a small team, a group of professionals, a whole hospital, or a vast monolithic organisation such as the NHS). Some, like Schein's definition, are more precise if somewhat long-winded:

> ... the pattern of shared basic assumptions – invented, discovered or developed by a given group as it learns to cope with its problems of external adaptation and internal integration – that has worked well enough to be considered valid and therefore to be taught to new members as the correct way to perceive, think and feel in relationship to those problems.[31]

The Schein definition has the benefit of capturing one of the basic challenges faced by any culture: to establish a common meaning and reconcile the often divergent aims and actions of its members.

Given the plethora and diversity of perspectives, a universally accepted definition of culture is unlikely ever to be achieved. But at the heart of many definitions is the view that culture comprises that which is shared and taken for granted between members of an organisation. That might include, for example, the beliefs, values, attitudes, habits, codes of practice, and social norms that guide working behaviour, as well as the routines, traditions, symbols, ceremonies, and rewards that underpin organisational life.[12,32] These shared ways of thinking and behaving help define what is legitimate and acceptable in a group setting. They act as the social and normative glue that binds people in collective enterprise.[29] Yet much of culture emerges from largely hidden assumptions, which makes it difficult to recognise once we are inside the culture – and harder still to study. As the Chinese proverb says: 'The fish is always the last to discover the sea.' Culture can be viewed as the sea within which we all swim in our various organisational environments.

Conventionally, the literature on organisational culture is divided into two broad streams: corporate culturist approaches and interpretive approaches, as set out in Table 1.[12,33.] The corporate culturist approach views culture as an *attribute* – something that an organisation *has*. Culture, according to this view, is an operational variable that can be isolated, described, and manipulated by leaders alongside other organisational variables (including strategy, structure, and incentives) to achieve wider organisational goals. For those who subscribe to this conceptualisation, culture is viewed as the exclusive property of managers who seek to assimilate among their staff clearly enunciated company values and norms. It is clear that much of the prescriptive advice aimed at healthcare organisations contained in the management literature and inquiry recommendations collude with the corporate culturist perspective. Here, emphasis is placed on creating desirable cultures through the organisational processes used to recruit, socialise, and reward employees.[34]

In contrast, interpretive approaches construe culture more holistically – as something that an organisation *is*. Here, culture serves as a metaphor for describing the organisation. Cast in this way, organisations are perceived as cultural *systems*, with culture something that penetrates every aspect and layer of an organisation.[11] This marks a shift from seeing culture as an isolatable variable to an understanding of culture as the context of all organisational variables. Interpretive approaches understand culture as something that arises spontaneously from social interaction and is actively lived, breathed, and shaped by all organisational members. The interpretive perspective helps to shed light on the limits of management control and offers fewer convenient levers for managers to shape employees' values for instrumental ends.

Table 1 Comparing corporate culturist and interpretive perspectives

	Corporate culturist	Interpretive
Disciplinary base	Popular management books, business self-help texts, and management consultancy.	Academic literature, including theoretical and empirical work within social anthropology, organisation studies, and industrial sociology.
Theory of cultural cohesion	Organisations are characterised by a single, homogenous culture that is consistent across all departments and levels.	Organisations are internally differentiated and comprise an array of coexisting and sometimes competing subcultures.
Theory of organisation	Organisations are objective, real entities that exist independently from organisation theory.	Organisations do not have an objective reality with members socially constructing multiple subjective realities.
Culture change agents	Culture change is a project that is led, organised, and controlled by managers to meet wider organisational objectives.	All members of an organisation are continuously involved in creating, changing, and reproducing culture.
Nature of culture change	Culture change is a planned and predetermined episodic event that is implemented and directed by managers.	Culture change cannot be assumed to follow managerially espoused values; rather, culture change arises spontaneously from everyday social interaction.

Significant as this cleavage in conceptions of organisational culture has been, the distinction between the two polarised approaches risks sustaining caricatured or simplistic positions – for instance, in relation to how easy (or not) it is to manipulate culture for managerial purposes. In an attempt to tread a middle ground between these two opposed camps, some researchers conceive organisational culture as something that is not so easily managed: instead, it is assumed, first, that its key characteristics can at least be described and assessed in terms of their functional contributions to broader managerial and organisational objectives; and second, once an understanding of these characteristics is attained, some shaping and moulding of these dynamics is possible.[11]

3.2 Layered Nature of Culture

Despite the often heated debates over the precise meaning of organisational culture, most commentators agree that it is layered in nature. A useful starting point for a discussion of the layering of culture is the framework proposed by the organisational psychologist Edgar Schein.[31] This distinguishes between three cultural levels.

- **Level 1: artefacts**. First and most tangible are the surface-level attributes that can be immediately seen, felt, and heard when one enters an organisation. In a healthcare facility, these might include the physical and social environment, including the layout of workspaces (e.g. open-plan or closed-plan offices), the spatial location of wards, staff rotas, job titles, and dress codes (think white coats as a symbol of doctors in the USA, but not the UK). They also include workplace rites, rituals, and ceremonies (e.g. induction programmes, retirement parties, and award dinners) that send explicit signals about what is important and affirm what the organisation stands for. Although artefacts are easy to observe, they may be more difficult to decipher, and it is particularly dangerous to try and infer their meaning without a knowledge of the deeper assumptions and beliefs on which they are based.
- **Level 2: beliefs and values**. Beliefs and values are part of the cognitive substructure of an organisational culture. They are the social principles and moral and ethical codes and standards that members believe have intrinsic worth. These are the largely unwritten rules used to justify particular behaviours, provide a rationale for choosing between alternate courses of action, and distinguish right from wrong. Relevant healthcare examples include beliefs around respect for patient autonomy and dignity and the beliefs that guide actions around speaking up and responding to concerns about professional transgressions and unsafe care.
- **Level 3: basic assumptions**. Deeper still, but much harder to access and observe, are the often unconscious and unexamined expectations, perceptions, and presuppositions shared by organisational members that underpin day-to-day work. In a healthcare delivery context, for example, these may include assumptions about the nature of the caring role or about hierarchies in clinical settings and respect (or otherwise) for the knowledge

and perspectives of patients and relatives. According to Schein, the essence of an organisation's culture lies at this level. However, in practical terms, basic assumptions are difficult to identify. As they are preconscious, they are also harder to openly challenge and modify.

A layered approach implies that understanding an organisation's culture requires examination of a very complex array of observable artefacts and the values, beliefs, and largely hidden unconscious assumptions that support them. Culture is often compared to an iceberg, with most of an organisation's beliefs and basic assumptions lying submerged beneath the surface and invisible to the naked eye.

Difficulties in interpreting an organisation's culture are compounded where an organisation's *espoused culture* – as reflected in official documentation such as mission statements, glossy corporate brochures, and the speeches of senior executives – contrasts with the *culture in practice* created routinely by employees and experienced by service users on a daily basis.[35] For example, in its publicity material and formal reports, the Mid Staffordshire NHS Foundation Trust espoused a strong commitment to providing patients with safe, high-quality, compassionate care. However, as the Francis inquiry concluded, the actual care experienced by many patients fell far short of this ideal.[21] Divergences between espoused cultures and cultures in practice may explain why so many organisational cultures appear paradoxical, and contradictory, both to employees and those they interact with.

3.3 Subcultures

The discussion so far has largely assumed that healthcare organisations are characterised by a single unitary culture. But is this the case? Corporate culturist approaches assume organisational unity, with managers setting the tone that organisational members follow. But many people familiar with complex and dynamic healthcare organisations will recognise that their cultures are usually far from uniform or coherent. Some cultural attributes may be visible across an organisation, but other cultural attributes may be prominent only in particular subcultures of that same organisation. Differences between these cultures can result in significant problems when attempting to facilitate intergroup communication, cooperation, and coordination. Different cultures may emerge, for example, within different occupational or professional groups or within teams working in physically separated spaces or faced with different temporal working patterns (e.g. night-shift workers). Differences in culture may also be linked to relative position within the organisational hierarchy and to professional roles. Nursing, for example, has traditionally had a much stricter disciplinary code and a more punitive approach to clinical errors than medicine. And cultural differences may be influenced by factors such as age cohort, gender, class, and ethnicity.

Subcultures are also likely to be associated with different levels of power and influence, whose dynamics may alter and shift over time. The traditional dominance of the medical culture in the NHS, for example, has been challenged in recent years by the rise of the management culture.[11] But despite the focus in the literature on top managers shaping culture, distinct and vivid subcultures are evident among non-management staff – such as ancillary staff, receptionists, porters, and cleaners. These subcultures may hold very different values and assumptions to those occupying more privileged positions at the apex of the organisation.

Differences between subcultures can result in significant problems when attempting to facilitate intergroup communication, cooperation, and coordination. Conflicts between cultural subgroups may reflect differences in power and legitimacy as well as outlook, and they can be as much about a struggle for expression of identity, meaning, and purpose as about competition for resources, autonomy, and control. For instance, healthcare professionals and managers may use the same language and terminology when speaking of patient care (relating to quality, safety, or the use of evidence, for example) but mean very different things and understand the proper solutions in very different ways. These conflicts can be difficult to manage because each subculture may have different values and established ways of working that sometimes are directly opposed to each other.[36] Indeed, a growing evidence base documents the subcultural diversity that exists within healthcare organisations and how, at different times, different subcultures may cooperate or compete (sometimes simultaneously) for organisational power, influence, status, and resources.[37–41]

3.3.1 Conceptualising Subcultures in Complex Organisations

Researchers have (broadly) adopted two complementary perspectives for understanding the role of organisational subcultures in complex organisations.

The first perspective is based on a framework that defines subcultures relative to an organisation's overall cultural patterns and, in particular, its dominant values as espoused by senior managers.[42] This framework presents three key types of subculture.

- **Enhancing subcultures** may develop in specialist work teams or units where individuals adhere closely to and amplify the values of the dominant management culture more fervently than those working in the rest of the organisation. Such enhancing subcultures can arise when special project groups are tasked and resourced with delivering transformational change, perhaps shaped by charismatic local leadership. They may also be a feature of healthcare organisations characterised by stable employment patterns, where long-serving employees are steeped in the traditions and values of an organisation.

- **Orthogonal subcultures** may arise in organisational subgroups whose members subscribe to both the values and beliefs of the dominant organisational culture, while simultaneously espousing and enacting their own professional values, which are influenced and shaped from outside the organisation. Many medical specialties and subspecialties in healthcare can be characterised in this way – for example, the traditional allegiance of clinicians to the royal colleges in the NHS.
- **Countercultures** are threats to the dominant culture and may arise in organisational enclaves that espouse values that challenge (overtly or covertly) the dominant culture of an organisation. For example, healthcare professionals with different tribal loyalties may seek to defend or develop their professional identities where there are pockets of clinical resistance to new management initiatives and diktats. It can sometimes be difficult to decide whether countercultures are stubborn resisters to necessary change, simply defenders of professional traditions, or perceptive opponents of damaging new directions.

The second (but complementary) perspective recognises that subcultures in healthcare organisations relate to department, ward, speciality, clinical network, and, most obviously, occupational group.[11] Occupational groups may in turn be subdivided into specialisms and services (e.g. radiology, anaesthetics, oncology, cardiology, etc.). In overlaying the basic occupational subculture, we might expect each specialism to elaborate its own distinctive subculture based on anatomical functions, diseases, complications, procedures, therapies, and the patient group it deals with.

Two of the major professional groupings involved in improving quality and safety – healthcare professionals and managers – may differ in a number of important regards in their group cultures. Humour, caricatures, and stereotypes may be invoked by either party to reinforce these divergences – for example, talk of 'going over to the dark side' when clinicians get involved in management. These cultural divergences have important implications for collaborative work, especially for individuals in hybrid roles who may either retain a cultural allegiance to their base group or seek to adopt the cultural orientations that are the norms for new roles. Thus, one challenge is to devise strategies on cultural transformation that successfully achieve a degree of cultural fit between these two key groups.

3.3.2 Organisational Culture As a Subculture

Organisational culture is itself a subculture within a larger set of supra-cultures, including the overall culture of the NHS and the national culture of the UK.[43] As healthcare becomes more global with regular movement of care staff across national borders, major shapers of the cultural aspects of care may also include different national, ethnic, or religious cultures. The NHS employs an increasingly diverse workforce and staff from other countries may bring very different values and beliefs regarding what constitutes good quality care, and this may influence the other staff with whom they collaborate.

In addition, healthcare professionals are socialised into various professional cultures, which may have an enduring and profound influence on working values and practices.[44] For example, nurses and doctors receive much of their formative socialisation through their professional training and engagements, rather than as a consequence of their organisational setting.[45–47] Public opinion, media reporting, and regulatory frameworks may also exert an influence on shaping internal culture. In summary, any exploration of healthcare culture needs to clarify which level of culture is to be examined and be alert to the influence of supra-cultures and subcultures. Making sense of this multilevel cultural mosaic in a complex professional bureaucracy such as a healthcare organisation should be an essential part of any cultural diagnosis prior to embarking on improvement.

4 Measuring and Assessing Culture

This section introduces some of the tools, instruments, and approaches for measuring and assessing cultures in healthcare organisations. We discuss some of the key challenges and questions around their use.

4.1 Tools, Instruments, and Approaches for Measuring and Assessing Cultures

The growing interest in understanding and shaping cultures in healthcare organisations has prompted development of practical tools and instruments to measure and assess organisational culture across a range of healthcare settings. Such tools are now widely used in the NHS and other health systems to support quality improvement.[48] But measuring and assessing organisational culture is far from straightforward.[49,50] What are the relative merits of a quantitative or qualitative approach to data gathering? How many respondents are required to represent the organisation as a whole – as well as its constituent subcultures? Should data be sought only from senior management or from a wider range of respondents? And what is the most cost-effective method of gathering data?

These questions have no definitive or clear-cut answers. Responses will depend on issues such as the definition of culture being used, who it is that wants to know about culture and for what purposes, what they are going to do with the information, what resources are available for the investigation, and so on. For example, qualitative and quantitative approaches are associated with different strengths and weaknesses, and choosing between the two can hinge on a trade-off between depth and breadth of data. Qualitative approaches may offer detailed insights while quantitative approaches allow for the examination of larger sample sizes. One way to harness the strengths of both approaches is to combine them. Yauch and Steudel[51] argue that cultural exploration should start with a period of qualitative assessment; the insights gained can then be used to select the most appropriate quantitative instrument and method of administration.

The diversity and contested nature of understanding about culture necessarily means that there are diverse and contested means of assessing it. The most comprehensive review on culture measurement has identified 70 methods suitable for exploring and assessing organisational culture in healthcare contexts, ranging from structured self-report questionnaires to projective techniques and emergent ethnographic approaches.[48] Unsurprisingly, the review found that most empirical and practical work in healthcare to date has focused more on understanding and assessing the first two cultural levels of Schein's framework[31] – level 1 (artefacts) and level 2 (beliefs and values) – rather than on uncovering the deep-seated and harder-to-reach aspects of organisational culture outlined under level 3 (see Section 3.2). The overall conclusion of the 2008 review by Mannion et al. is that there is no such thing as an ideal instrument or approach for assessing organisational cultures and that an instrument that works well in one context may be inappropriate in another.[48] Different instruments have various uses and offer different insights: they may reveal some areas and aspects of an organisation's culture but obscure others. Box 2 presents three examples of culture assessment tools used in healthcare organisations.

Box 2 THREE EXAMPLES OF CULTURE ASSESSMENT TOOLS USED IN HEALTHCARE

ORGANISATIONS

The **Safety Attitudes Questionnaire (SAQ)** is a major summative (quantitative) assessment tool developed in the USA by Sexton et al.[52] It is now widely used in the UK NHS to help organisations assess their safety culture and track changes over time.[53] The SAQ is a reworking and refinement of a similar tool widely used in the aviation industry. Various versions of the SAQ exist, typically comprising some 60 survey items using five-point Likert scales in six safety-related domains: safety climate, teamwork, stress recognition, perceptions of management, working conditions, and job satisfaction. Completed by individuals, scores are then aggregated to give an indication of the overall strength of the organisation's extant safety culture. The SAQ tool has been adapted for use in a range of healthcare settings, including primary care, nursing homes, long-term care facilities, and intensive care units.[54]

The **Manchester Patient Safety Framework (MaPSaF)** is a facilitative (qualitative) educational tool developed by academic colleagues at the University of Manchester.[55] It aims to provide insight into safety culture and how it can be improved among teams and organisations. Exploring nine dimensions of patient safety, the tool describes what an organisation would look like at different levels of maturity in relation to patient safety, ranging from 'pathological' (why do we waste our time on patient safety issues?) to 'generative' (managing patient safety is an integral part of everything we do). Assessment is carried out in facilitator-led workshops. The assessments can be used to prompt reflections, stimulate discussions, and understand strengths and weaknesses. Although the framework was originally developed for use in the primary care sector, it has since been adapted for use in other healthcare settings.[56]

The **Culture of Care Barometer (CCB)** is a diagnostic tool designed and developed by Rafferty et al. at King's College London[57] to help healthcare organisations measure the culture of care they provide and explore certain areas of culture in greater depth. A self-assessment tool, the barometer can be used to stimulate reflection and prompt discussion and understanding of the culture of care at different levels in an organisation. A five-point Likert scale is used to indicate strength of agreement with 30 questions, which can be grouped into four broad dimensions related to supporting the delivery of high-quality care: the resources to deliver quality care; the support needed to do a good job; a worthwhile job that offers the chance to develop; and the opportunity to improve team working.

4.2 Assessing the Relationship between Culture, Quality, and Performance

Establishing links between culture, quality, and performance through research is not an easy task. A 2003 review concluded that evidence for an association between culture and performance in healthcare contexts was weak, with a number of claims based on methodologically poor research.[58] The most recent systematic review of work in this area, based on 62 studies, found a 'consistently positive association between culture and outcomes across multiple studies, settings, and countries'.[59] Most studies included in the review were quantitative (94%) and cross-sectional (81%); only four studies were classified as intervention studies and none was a randomised controlled trial.

Some studies have found positive associations between organisational culture and a range of quality-related phenomena, including the implementation of quality systems in hospitals,[60] attitudes to and satisfaction with the use of clinical information systems,[61] hospital performance,[62] cost containment,[63] and staff engagement.[64] Almost three-quarters of studies in the 2017 review reported an association between a positive culture (as defined in the study) and favourable patient outcomes; the other studies showed either no association or, in some cases, contradictory findings. However, the evidence base generally is problematic. Difficulties in establishing the direction of causality between culture and outcomes are evident. There are also concerns about the degree of separation between independent and dependent variables in some of the studies. It is questionable, for example, whether it is appropriate to assess the effect of espoused values on employee loyalty and commitment when loyalty and commitment are values themselves.[65]

Similarly, difficult is demonstrating the impact of efforts to engineer changes in organisational culture. The only published systematic review of intervention studies 'did not identify any effective strategies to change organisational culture'.[66] One high-profile study of an intervention (the Safer Patients Initiative) with a controlled design found that although there was a small improvement in staff attitudes to organisational culture in intervention hospitals, the initiative had no significant effect on patient safety outcomes (as measured by prescription errors, adverse events, and mortality rates).[67]

Numerous empirical research studies suggest that there is no single *best* culture that is always associated with successful outcomes across a range of organisational dimensions. Rather, organisational culture seems to be linked to quality and performance in a contingent manner, with those aspects of quality and performance that are most valued within the dominant culture being the aspects on which the organisation performs best.[11]

An early study in Canadian, UK, and US hospitals[65] found, for example, that hospitals with inwardly oriented cultures that emphasised managing through informal, interpersonal relationships performed significantly above average on measures of employee loyalty and commitment. In contrast, those with more outward-looking cultures and procedural management performed better on measures of external stakeholder satisfaction. A later study based on large-scale longitudinal research across all English NHS hospital trusts[62] replicated some of these findings, suggesting that the specific domains of performance that are valued within a dominant culture are those in which the hospitals performed best. The key implication of these findings – from a management perspective at least – is the need to develop cultures in healthcare organisations that are aligned with key policy objectives in the NHS. In addition, the appropriateness or otherwise of extant cultures needs to be regularly reviewed and revitalised to prevent a strategic drift between extant cultures and shifting priorities in the wider environment.

Any links between culture and performance or quality in a healthcare context are likely to be highly contingent, complex, and non-linear, making it inherently difficult to draw hard-and-fast or generalisable recommendations that apply across diverse healthcare contexts.[68] One key difficulty lies in disentangling the direction of causality between culture and quality or performance. Although most attention to date has centred on how culture may affect performance, it is equally plausible that certain cultures arise from high-performing organisations. That is, performance drives culture. More likely still is that culture and performance are recursive, mutually constituted, and reinforcing, and dependent on wider contexts and influences. Indeed, the widely used phrase 'the way things are done around here' could be interpreted as being as much a definition of performance as it is of culture. Box 3 presents a summary of some of the cultural characteristics of high-performing and low-performing NHS hospital trusts, based on a number of case studies.

Box 3 CULTURAL CHARACTERISTICS OF HIGH-PERFORMING AND LOW-PERFORMING NHS HOSPITAL TRUSTS[11,69]

Detailed, qualitative case-study work in the English NHS has helped to shed light on the managerial cultural characteristics of high-performing and low-performing NHS hospital trusts.

Mannion et al.'s study found very different cultural patterning across high-performing and low-performing hospitals, and these suggest areas where managerial action may usefully be directed. In particular, strong information-based systems of accountability, empowered middle management, and pro-performance values all seem to be important underpinnings of a clearly articulated corporate strategy. These foundations in turn highlight the importance of contingent leadership – that is, leadership that is able to express and embody corporate vision, but equally able to follow through with the transactional details. For example, high-performing trusts were characterised by top-down, command-and-control styles of leadership, with the management setting clear and explicit performance objectives for the trust and establishing robust internal monitoring arrangements to support these aims.

Although the high-performing trusts had a long history of strong top-down styles of leadership, it was clear that the limits of this approach were appreciated and more devolved systems of leadership and governance were being implemented. In contrast, low-performing trusts were characterised by leaders, in particular chief executives, who were generally regarded as lacking the transactional skills required to develop and maintain robust systems of performance management. Many of the senior management regimes at the low-performing trusts were described as being remote and disconnected from day-to-day issues in the wider organisation. Terms such as 'clique' and 'inner circle' were widely used in these trusts to describe the virtual separation and sometimes self-regarding nature of the senior management teams. Moreover, in the low-performing trusts, loyalty to the leadership group was the dominant cultural trait, with whistleblowing or questioning of senior management decisions the ultimate taboo.

5 Making Culture Change Happen

5.1 Strategies for Managing Culture Change

In popular management books (such as those discussed in Section 2), it is often assumed that by using the right strategies, senior management can change, manage, or manipulate organisational culture to beneficial organisational ends. An alternative perspective is that organisational members do not always respond predictably to these efforts. They may even be resistant to top-down efforts to change organisational values, assumptions, and beliefs that underpin ways of working. Since a basic function of organisational culture is to provide a stable and durable platform for a way of living and working, it is small wonder that even modest changes to a working culture may stall or may perhaps provoke apparently disproportionate reactions of anger and resistance. A diverse range of conceptual frameworks and models for understanding the stages of culture change can be found in the literature.[12,70] Despite some significant differences between them, the models share some common elements and areas of focus:

- **crises** as a trigger for significant organisational change. A crisis may result in rapid swings in organisational norms and established patterns of working – for example, the need to rapidly introduce news ways of working in response to challenges posed by the COVID-19 pandemic. In other contexts, it is not unheard of for managers to talk up or even instigate a crisis in order to stimulate and justify culture change
- **leadership** in detecting the need for change and shaping that change by recognising the nature of the problem to be addressed, establishing new roles and responsibilities, and mediating in conflict situations
- **re-learning and re-education** as a means of embedding and helping to explain the assimilation of new cultures and the search for new cultural possibilities
- **success** to consolidate the new order and counter natural resistance to change. As one of the key functions of organisational culture is to establish and stabilise ways of organising and interacting, resistance is inherent to any culture change efforts.

A necessary first step in developing a culture change strategy is the decision to target either 'first order' or 'second order' change.[70]

- During first order change, the focus is on evolutionary growth (more of the same, but better) with the aim of retaining and building on those established values, traditions, and working practices that have served the organisation well over a period of years.
- In contrast, second order change (creating something different to achieve a radical break with the past) is often used in response to a growing crisis or deficiency in the existing culture. It involves something that cannot be addressed adequately by a change *in* culture but rather demands a fundamental change *of* culture. The focus is on nurturing radically new values and ways of working within the organisation.

It is plausible that the more radical a proposed shift in the content of a culture, the greater resistance to change will be. For example, an attempt to change the professional values and beliefs that have been affirmed over many decades and are tightly interwoven into the fabric of clinical practice is likely to be met with greater organisational resistance than minor modifications to corporate arte-facts, such as new company logos, re-designed mission statements, and other similar changes.

In most organisations, especially in complex and dynamic healthcare settings, such sharp distinctions between first order and second order change may be difficult to delineate, and a succession of small, incremental changes may ultimately lead to large-scale, radical change. In practice, most organisational change will require a judicious balance between transformation and continuity while seeking to avoid the introduction of new dysfunctions. The challenge, therefore, is to remain faithful to those aspects of the culture that have served the organisation well in the past, while identifying the cultural aspects that need to be reformed or replaced.

5.2 Potential Levers and Influences on Organisations' Ability to Manage Culture Change

As we have seen, there is an absence of robust evidence to guide culture change. This has not prevented commentators from identifying a range of factors that influence the ability of organisations to manage a cultural shift. [50,70] The key levers and influences described in the literature are discussed in the following subsections.

5.2.1 Organisational Structures

Organisational structure is the way in which work is organised into functional or operational units. Culture flows in and around these formal structures and is shaped by how they work. Structures therefore represent the framework in which relations are formed, with particular structures fostering particular sets of working practices and making others more problematic. [12] For example, a hospital with a strong hierarchical structure and steep vertical reporting lines may inhibit attempts to promote horizontal, cross-departmental working. In comparison, a highly decentralised organisation which devolves power and resources to semi-autonomous units may find it more difficult to develop common corporate values and ways of working. Some would argue that to be successful, a culture change programme should take heed of the existing organisational structure and understand how this shapes and sustains local working practices. [12] In some organisations, a realignment of existing structures may be an effective way of engendering wider culture change via the impact it has on disturbing established patterns of interaction and communication in an organisation.

5.2.2 Ensuring Alignment with the External Context

In conducting a culture change programme, it may be important to adjust the alignment or fit between a culture and the wider environment. As changes in the external environment occur, so must the internal culture change if it is not to become obsolete. This adaptive approach necessarily requires an assessment of cultural lag or strategic drift to gauge the gap between the culture in use and the required culture. The public context of the NHS has changed dramatically over the past two decades, and some advocate that it is important that the organisation responds to these changes.[21] This perspective puts the issue of adaptability at the top of the agenda in discussions of organisational health and effectiveness.[70]

5.2.3 Adopting an Appropriate Leadership Style

Leaders play an important role in creating, embedding, and transmitting desirable cultural attributes. Research has shown that a range of styles of leadership is important for beneficial organisational functioning across different healthcare contexts.[11] Based on empirical work, several specific strategies to create positive cultures have been advocated for senior leaders in healthcare organisations.[71,72] These include:

- continually reinforcing an inspiring vision of the work of their organisations
- promoting staff health and well-being
- listening to staff and encouraging them to be involved in decision-making, problem-solving, and innovation at all levels
- providing staff with helpful feedback on how they are doing and celebrating good performance
- taking effective, supportive action to address system problems and other challenges when improvement is needed
- developing and modelling excellent teamwork
- making sure that staff feel safe, supported, respected, and valued at work.

Box 4 highlights the findings of an evaluation of a culture change initiative that focused on the role of leadership in promoting positive changes.

BOX 4 LEADING POSITIVE CULTURE CHANGE IN HOSPITAL SETTINGS[73]

A 2018 evaluation of a culture change initiative (Leadership Saves Lives) in the USA focused on leadership actions to promote positive changes in organisational culture in 10 hospitals.

The initiative involved fostering improvements in five areas of organisational culture thought to be related to hospital performance: learning environment, senior management support, psychological safety, commitment to the organisation, and time for improvement.

The evaluation found that changes in culture over a two-year period varied substantially between hospitals. The experience of the 'guiding coalitions' (multidisciplinary teams specifically created to guide the collaborative efforts in each hospital) differed markedly across hospitals. In the hospitals that achieved substantial and positive shifts in culture, the following characteristics were evident:

- representation of staff from different disciplines and levels in the organisational hierarchy
- authentic participation and engagement of diverse perspectives in the work of the guiding coalition
- distinct patterns of managing conflict, fatigue, and motivation over time.

Hospitals with marked positive shifts in culture (measured by a validated 31-item questionnaire) also experienced significant decreases in risk-standardised mortality rates (in this case for treatment of acute myocardial infarction).

An important lesson from this study is that hospital cultures may have some sort of impact on the work of clinical teams and departments and, in turn, on the quality and outcome of care given to patients. The approach taken by senior managers and leaders does, therefore, appear to matter. These findings give clues as to what elements of culture need attention from hospital leaders and boards. These include, but are not limited to:

- fostering a learning environment
- offering sustained and visible senior management support to clinical teams and services
- ensuring that staff across the organisation feel 'psychologically safe' and able to speak up when things are felt to be going wrong.

5.2.4 The Ability to Create a Sense of Ownership

Many employees in an organisation will have a high personal stake in maintaining the prevailing order. A change often invokes a sense of loss and anxiety, and reactions to change can be unpredictable and diverse. Even a few disaffected individuals can cause disruption and block reform. Vestiges of the old culture can prevail and thwart efforts at reform if they hold positions of power, creating obstacles to redesigning services and nurturing new values and working practices. Addressing these challenges may involve creating a critical mass of employees who buy into a culture change programme as well as opposing those who may seek to hold back reform.

Successful cultural change, then, requires political skills and the management of organisational politics.[28]

5.2.5 Managing External Influences

Outside interests may sometimes support or alternatively cut across and work against efforts towards internal cultural reform. Culture change strategies therefore need be alert to the potential opportunities and constraints posed by external stakeholders in shaping the values and behaviour of healthcare professionals. For example, the government's approach to naming and shaming poorly performing trusts may be detrimental to attempts by trusts to develop no-blame cultures in which employees feel comfortable reporting errors.[70] Moreover, any attempts to change organisational culture may also need to target powerful and influential external bodies such as the royal colleges, which exert control over training and, through early socialisation, influence the internalisation of core professional values and ways of working.

5.2.6 Identifying and Responding to Dysfunctional Consequences

Unintended and dysfunctional consequences of culture change strategies frequently arise. The capacity to identify and react to these consequences is an imperative in managing change. For example, although the rise of performance measurement cultures in the NHS linked to new systems of checking, verification, and audit have been associated with substantial improvements in quality of care, they have nevertheless induced a range of adverse consequences for organisations, staff, and patients.[74]

5.2.7 Aligning Cognitive and Behavioural Change

Cultural change strategies can give rise to at least three different organisational outcomes.[12]

First, change arising at the level of individual cognition (e.g. the values and beliefs that healthcare professionals hold around person-centred care) but with no corresponding change in behaviour. This may occur when employees align with the espoused principle but in practice find it difficult to adopt new ways of working.

Second, change at the behavioural level may not always be matched by change at the cognitive level if the beliefs underpinning working practices are largely unaffected. This is possible when, for example, compliance with a new top-down and imposed clinical framework is enforced by rules and the threat of sanctions, but does not affect the underlying, intrinsic motivation and commitment of staff.

Finally, there can be change at both the behavioural and cognitive levels. Some commentators argue that this is likely to result in the most self-sustaining form of change because employees genuinely value the new ways of working and behaviours become thoroughly embedded and routinised. The corollary is that to sustain long-term change, strategies should helpfully aim to influence *both* deeper changes in thinking as well as surface-level manifestations.[12]

6 Conclusions

Culture may indeed lie at the root of many of the service failings of complex organisations. Conversely, it may also be key to improving quality and safety. Despite its ubiquity as a diagnosis and prescription, culture remains an elusive concept fraught with competing interpretations and difficult to pin down with any degree of precision. Too often, culture is used by policymakers and managers as a prescriptive catch-all, used to explain everything – and consequently nothing. And despite the growing number of approaches, frameworks, and tools available to inform culture change at different levels in healthcare systems and organisations, closer probing of the literature suggests that the supporting evidence base is still rather thin – to the extent that in many areas, empirical data are largely absent. This, in turn, suggests that a more sober assessment of the task of cultural transformation in healthcare is warranted. There remains a challenging policy-focused research agenda to uncover the ingredients of successful culture change.

Substantive areas that warrant further and more sustained attention include the following.

First, although much of this Element has sought to unpack culture, we also need to take a differentiated and more nuanced view of healthcare quality, safety, and improvement. So, the challenge becomes one of developing a new understanding of which components of culture might influence which aspects of performance, and of how promising change might be sought in these areas. This is an altogether more complex and nuanced approach than undifferentiated demands for cultural transformation.

Second, healthcare cultures are co-produced by interactions with other players. Patients, carers, relatives, and other health service stakeholders (e.g. social care workers, service commissioners, and regulators) may all be important in shaping prevailing local cultures as they interact with those delivering services. Thus, future studies of healthcare culture may need to embrace a much wider range of participants and perspectives than has been the norm in culture studies.

Third, cultural change requires political skills involving the successful management of micro-organisational politics and partisan subcultural interests.

Empirical studies and theoretical frameworks that shed light on how health-care organisations can become more open and receptive to a wide diversity of voices, and which build a broad consensus around the cultural destinations sought and the mechanisms that will carry organisations towards these destinations, may be key to unlocking sustained change in a politically infused institution such as the NHS.

Finally, there is a real need for more and better-tested bespoke instruments, tools, and approaches for diagnosing, measuring, and assessing healthcare cultures. Given the dynamic nature and complexity of culture in healthcare contexts, the building, testing, and refining of a variety of such tools and approaches will be an ongoing task.

Culture is a useful lens when managing and understanding processes of change in complex healthcare organisations. But simplistic attempts to manage or engineer culture change from above, based on old ideas from the 1980s, airport bestsellers, are unlikely to succeed. Efforts to make a change need to be sensitive to the complexity and highly stratified nature of culture in and across NHS organisations. Of particular concern is the need to be alert to the role of local subcultures, which at different times may be driving forces for change, defenders of the status quo (for good or ill), or covert countercultures quietly undermining necessary reforms. This is not to argue that managers have no influence on shaping healthcare cultures; managing with a cultural awareness, rather than managing culture per se, may be a realistic goal.

7 Further Reading

This section suggests further reading for those who want to find out more about culture and cultural change in organisations, including healthcare cultures specifically, and the relationships between culture and patient outcomes.

- Mannion and Davies[68] – overview of the ways in which culture is linked to quality in healthcare organisations that draws on theory and empirical evidence.
- Braithwaite et al.[59] – systematic review and synthesis of the evidence on the extent to which organisational and workplace cultures are associated with patient outcomes.
- Department of Health[15] – report reviewing the scale and nature of failures in NHS healthcare and which identifies organisational systems and cultures as key components of health system redesign.
- Institute of Medicine[13] – sets a national agenda for reducing medical health errors and improving patient safety through the design of a safer health system.

- Francis[21] – report of the Mid Staffordshire NHS Foundation Trust public inquiry, which details serious systemic failings in care at the Trust, discusses the role of organisational culture, and suggests recommendations for change.
- Mannion et al.[11] – textbook that introduces theories from a wide range of disciplines and sets out definitions of cultures and performance, looking in particular at specific characteristics that help or hinder performance, and includes case studies of hospital trusts and primary care trusts.
- Martin[28] – textbook that offers an interdisciplinary overview of the organisational culture literature and looks at the ways in which researchers have disagreed on questions of definitions, theoretical approaches, ideologies, and methods.
- Peters and Waterman[5] – bestselling example from the 1980s management handbook trend, which includes descriptions of the eight basic principles of management deemed to be essential for a successful organisation.
- Schein[31] – often considered a field-defining management book, it considers definitions of culture, the structure of culture, and the interrelationship between organisational culture and leadership.

Contributors

Conflicts of Interest

None.

Acknowledgements

The author thanks the peer reviewers for their insightful comments and recommendations to improve the Element. A list of peer reviewers is published at www.cambridge.org/IQ-peer-reviewers.

Funding

This Element was funded by THIS Institute (The Healthcare Improvement Studies Institute, www.thisinstitute.cam.ac.uk). THIS Institute is strengthening the evidence base for improving the quality and safety of healthcare. THIS Institute is supported by a grant to the University of Cambridge from the Health Foundation – an independent charity committed to bringing about better health and healthcare for people in the UK.

About the Author

Russell Mannion is Professor of Health Systems at the University of Birmingham, where he has held the Chair in Health Systems since 2010. He is Honorary Professor at the Australian Institute of Health Innovation, Macquarie University, and a Fellow of Bocconi University.

Creative Commons Licence

References

1. Williams R. *Keywords: A Vocabulary of Culture and Society*. New York: Oxford University Press; 1983.
2. Wright S. 'Culture' in anthropology and organizational studies. In: Wright S, editor. *Anthropology of Organizations*. London: Routledge; 1994: 1–31.
3. Jaques E. *The Changing Culture of a Factory*. London: Tavistock; 1951.
4. Pettigrew AM. On studying organisational cultures. *Adm Sci Q* 1979; 24: 570–81. https://doi.org/10.2307/2392363.
5. Peters T, Waterman RH. *In Search of Excellence: Lessons from America's Best-Run Companies*. New York: Harper and Row; 1982.
6. Deal T, Kennedy A. *Corporate Cultures: The Rites and Rituals of Corporate Life*. Harmondsworth: Penguin; 1982.
7. Abegglen JC, Stalk G. *Kaisha, the Japanese Corporation: The New Competitors in World Business*. New York: Basic Books; 1985.
8. Ohmae K. *The Mind of the Strategist: The Art of Japanese Business*. New York: McGraw-Hill; 1982.
9. Ouchi W. *Theory Z: How American Business Can Meet the Japanese Challenge*. Reading, MA: Addison Wesley; 1981.
10. Krepps DM. Corporate culture and economic theory. In: Alt JE, Shepsle KA, editors. *Perspectives on Positive Political Economy*. Cambridge: Cambridge University Press; 1990: 90–142. https://doi.org/10.1017/CBO9780511571657.
11. Mannion R, Davies HTO, Marshall MN. *Cultures for Performance in Health Care*. Maidenhead: Open University Press; 2005.
12. Brown A. *Organizational Culture*. London: Pitman; 1995.
13. Institute of Medicine. *To Err Is Human: Building a Safer Health System*. Washington, DC: National Academies Press; 1999. www.ncbi.nlm.nih.gov/books/NBK225182 (accessed 16 August 2021).
14. Institute of Medicine. *Crossing the Quality Chasm: A New Health System for the 21st Century*. Washington, DC: National Academies Press; 2001. www.ncbi.nlm.nih.gov/books/NBK222274 (accessed 30 March 2022).
15. Department of Health. *An Organisation with a Memory. Report of an Expert Working Group on Learning from Adverse Events in the NHS Chaired by the Chief Medical Officer*. London: Stationery Office; 2000. https://psnet.ahrq.gov/issue/organisation-memory-report-expert-group-learning-adverse-events-nhs-chaired-chief-medical (accessed 16 August 2021).

16. Boaden R. Quality improvement: theory and practice. *Br J Healthcare Manage* 2009; 15: 12–6. https://doi.org/10.12968/bjhc.2009.15.1.37892.

17. Ivers N, Foy R. Audit, feedback, and behaviour change. In: Dixon-Woods M, Brown K, Marjanovic S, et al., editors. *Elements of Improving Quality and Safety in Healthcare*. Cambridge: Cambridge University Press; forthcoming.

18. Radnor Z, Williams S. Lean and associated techniques for process improvement. In: Dixon-Woods M, Brown K, Marjanovic S, et al., editors. *Elements of Improving Quality and Safety in Healthcare*. Cambridge: Cambridge University Press; forthcoming.

19. Martin G, Dixon-Woods M. Collaboration-based approaches. In: Dixon-Woods M, Brown K, Marjanovic S, et al., editors. *Elements of Improving Quality and Safety in Healthcare*. Cambridge: Cambridge University Press; 2022. https://doi.org/10.1017/9781009236867.

20. Kennedy I. *Learning from Bristol: The Report of the Public Inquiry into Children's Heart Surgery at the Bristol Royal Infirmary 1984-1995*. 2001: CM 5207. https://webarchive.nationalarchives.gov.uk/ukgwa/20090811143758/www.bristol-inquiry.org.uk/index.htm (accessed 30 March 2022).

21. Francis R. *Report of the Mid Staffordshire NHS Foundation Trust Public Inquiry*. London: The Stationery Office; 2013. www.gov.uk/government/publications/report-of-the-mid-staffordshire-nhs-foundation-trust-public-inquiry (accessed 30 March 2022).

22. Gosport Independent Panel. *Gosport War Memorial Hospital: The Report of the Gosport Independent Panel*. London: HMSO; 2018: HC1084. www.gosportpanel.independent.gov.uk/panel-report (accessed 16 August 2021).

23. Davies H, Mannion R. Will prescriptions for cultural change improve the NHS? *BMJ* 2013; 346: f1305. https://doi.org/10.1136/bmj.f1305.

24. Goodwin N. NHS Inquiries and the problem of culture. *Polit Q* 2019; 90: 202–9. https://doi.org/10.1111/1467-923X.12693

25. Berwick D. *A Promise to Learn – A Commitment to Act: Improving the Safety of Patient Safety in England*. London: HMSO; 2013. www.gov.uk/government/publications/berwick-review-into-patient-safety (accessed 30 March 2022).

26. Powell M, Mannion R. 'Groundhog Day': The Coalition Government's Quality and Safety Reforms. In: Exworthy M, Mannion R, Powell M, editors. *Dismantling the NHS: Evaluating the Impact of Health Reforms*. Bristol: Policy Press; 2016: 323–42. https://doi.org/10.1332/policypress/9781447330226.001.0001.

27. Dixon-Woods M, Campbell A, Martin G, et al. Improving employee voice about transgressive or disruptive behavior: a case study. *Acad Med* 2019; 94: 579–85. http://doi.org/10.1097/ACM.0000000000002447.

28. Martin J. *Organizational Culture: Mapping the Terrain*. London: SAGE; 2002. https://dx.doi.org/10.4135/9781483328478.

29. Alvesson M. *Understanding Organizational Culture*. London: SAGE; 2013. https://dx.doi.org/10.4135/9781446280072.

30. Ott JS. *The Organizational Culture Perspective*. Pacific Grove: Brooks/ Cole; 1989.

31. Schein EH. *Organizational Culture and Leadership*. San Francisco: Jossey Bass; 1995.

32. Ehrhart MG, Schneider B, Macey WH. *Organizational Climate and Culture: An Introduction to Theory, Research, and Practice*. New York: Routledge; 2014.

33. Hatch MJ, Cunliffe AL. *Organization Theory: Modern Symbolic and Postmodern Perspectives, 2nd ed*. Oxford: Oxford University Press; 2006.

34. Denison R. *Corporate Culture and Organizational Effectiveness*. New York: Wiley; 1990.

35. Argyris C, Schon DA. *Theory in Practice*. San Francisco: Jossey Bass; 1978.

36. Martin J. *Cultures in Organizations: Three Perspectives*. Oxford: Oxford University Press; 1992.

37. Kitchener M. Mobilizing the logic of managerialism in professional fields: the case of academic health centre mergers. *Organ Stud* 2002; 23: 391–420. https://doi.org/10.1177/0170840602233004.

38. Evetts J. Short note: the sociology of professional groups: new directions. *Curr Sociol* 2006; 54: 133–43. https://doi.org/10.1177/0011392106057161.

39. Mannion R, Brown S, Beck M, Lunt N. Managing cultural diversity in healthcare partnerships: the case of LIFT. *J Health Organ Manage* 2011; 25: 645–57. https://doi.org/10.1108/14777261111178538.

40. Ovseiko PV, Melham K, Fowler J, Buchan AM. Organisational culture and post-merger integration in an academic health centre: a mixed-methods study. *BMC Health Serv Res* 2015; 15: 201–9. https://doi.org/10.1186 /s12913-014-0673-3.

41. Nembhard IM, Singer S, Shortell S, Rittenhouse D, Casalino L. The cultural complexity of medical groups. *Health Care Manage Rev* 2012; 37: 200–13. https://doi.org/10.1097/HMR.0b013e31822f54cd.

42. Martin J, Siehl C. Organizational culture and counterculture: an uneasy symbiosis. *Organ Dyn* 1983; 12: 52–4. https://doi.org/10.1016/0090-2616 (83)90033-5.

43. Nelson RE, Gopalan S. Do organizational cultures replicate national cultures? Isomorphism, rejection and reciprocal opposition in the corporate values of three countries. *Organ Stud* 2003; 24: 1115–51. https://doi.org/10.1177/01708406030247006.

44. Mannion R, Davies H, Powell M, et al. Healthcare scandals and the failings of doctors: do official inquiries hold the profession to account? *J Health Organ Manage* 2019; 33: 221–40. https://doi.org/10.1108/JHOM-04-2018-0126.

45. Glouberman S, Mintzberg H. Managing the care of health and the cure of disease – part I: differentiation. *Health Care Manage Rev* 2001; 26: 56–69. https://doi.org/10.1097/00004010-200101000-00006.

46. Glouberman S, Mintzberg H. Managing the care of health and the cure of disease – part II: integration. *Health Care Manage Rev* 2001; 26: 70–84. https://doi.org/10.1097/00004010-200101000-00007.

47. Horowitz R. *In the Public Interest: Medical Licensing and the Disciplinary Process.* New Brunswick, NJ: Rutgers University Press; 2012.

48. Mannion R, Davies H, Konteh F, et al. *Measuring and Assessing Organisational Culture in the NHS (OC1).* London: National Co-ordinating Centre for the National Institute for Health Research Service Delivery and Organisation Programme; 2008. https://njl-admin.nihr.ac.uk/document/download/2027506 (accessed 30 March 2022).

49. Jung T, Scott T, Davies HTO, et al. Instruments for exploring organizational culture: a review of the literature. *Publ Admin Rev* 2009; 69: 1087–96. https://doi.org/10.1111/j.1540-6210.2009.02066.x.

50. Scott T, Mannion R, Davies HTO, Marshall M. Implementing culture change in health care: theory and practice. *Int J Qual Health Care* 2003; 15: 111–8. https://doi.org/10.1093/intqhc/mzg021.

51. Yauch CA, Steudel HJ. Complementary use of qualitative and quantitative cultural assessment methods. *Organ Res Methods* 2003; 6: 465–81. https://doi.org/10.1177/1094428103257362.

52. Sexton JB, Helmreich RL, Neilands TB, et al. The safety attitudes questionnaire: psychometric properties, benchmarking data, and emerging research. *BMC Health Serv Res* 2006; 6: 44. https://doi.org/10.1186/1472-6963-6-44.

53. Mannion R, Konteh FH, Davies HTO. Assessing organisational culture for quality and safety improvement: a national survey of tools and tool use. *Qual Saf Health Care* 2009; 18: 153–6. http://dx.doi.org/10.1136/qshc.2007.024075.

54. Mesarić J, Šimić D, Katić M, et al. The safety attitudes questionnaire for out-of-hours service in primary healthcare – psychometric properties of the Croatian version. *PLoS One* 2020; 15: e0242065. https://doi.org/10.1371/journal.pone.0242065.

55. Kirk S, Parker D, Claridge T, Esmail A, Marshall M. Patient safety culture in primary care: developing a theoretical framework for practical use. *Qual Saf Health Care* 2007; 16: 313–20. http://dx.doi.org/10.1136/qshc.2006.018366.

56. Parker D. Managing risk in healthcare: understanding your safety culture using the Manchester Patient Safety Framework (MaPSaF). *J Nurs Manag* 2009; 17: 218–22. https://doi.org/10.1111/j.1365-2834.2009.00993.x.

57. Rafferty AM, Philippou J, Fitzpatrick JM, Pike G, Ball J. Development and testing of the 'Culture of Care Barometer' (CoCB) in healthcare organisations: a mixed methods study. *BMJ Open* 2017; 7: e016677. http://dx.doi.org/10.1136/bmjopen-2017-016677.

58. Scott T, Mannion R, Marshall M, Davies H. Does organisational culture influence health care performance? A review of the evidence. *J Health Serv Res Policy* 2003; 8: 105–17. https://doi.org/10.1258/135581903321466085.

59. Braithwaite J, Herkes J, Ludlow K, Testa L, Lamprell G. Association between organisational and workplace cultures, and patient outcomes: systematic review. *BMJ Open* 2017; 7: e017708. http://dx.doi.org/10.1136/bmjopen-2017-017708.

60. Shortell S, Jones R, Rademaker AW, et al. Assessing the impact of total quality management and organizational culture on multiple outcomes of care for coronary artery bypass graft surgery patients. *Med Care* 2000; 38: 207–17. https://doi.org/10.1097/00005650-200002000-00010.

61. Callen JL, Braithwaite J, Westbrook JI. The importance of medical and nursing sub-cultures in the implementation of clinical information systems. *Meth Inform Med* 2009; 48: 196–202. https://doi.org/10.3414/ME9212.

62. Jacobs R, Mannion R, Davies HTO, et al. The relationship between organizational culture and performance in acute hospitals. *Soc Sci Med* 2013; 76: 115–25. https://doi.org/10.1016/j.socscimed.2012.10.014.

63. Zhou P, Bundorf K, Le Chang J, Xue D. Organizational culture and its relationship with hospital performance in public hospitals in China. *Health Serv Res* 2011; 46: 2139–60. https://doi.org/10.1111/j.1475-6773.2011.01336.x.

64. Fedorowsky R, Peles-Bortz A, Masarwa S, et al. Carbapenem-resistant Enterobacteriaceae carriers in acute care hospitals and postacute-care facilities: the effect of organizational culture on staff attitudes, knowledge,

practices, and infection acquisition rates. *Am J Infect Control* 2015; 43: 935–9. https://doi.org/10.1016/j.ajic.2015.05.014.

65. Gerowitz MB, Lemieux-Charles L, Heginbothan C, Johnson B. Top management culture and performance in Canadian, UK and US hospitals. *Health Serv Manage Res* 1996; 9: 69–78. https://doi.org/10.1177/095148489600900201.

66. Parmelli E, Flodgren G, Beyer F, et al. The effectiveness of strategies to change organisational culture to improve healthcare performance: a systematic review. *Implement Sci* 2011; 6: 33. https://doi.org/10.1186/1748-5908-6-33.

67. Benning A, Ghaleb M, Suokas A, et al. Large scale organisational intervention to improve patient safety in four UK hospitals: mixed method evaluation. *BMJ* 2011; 342: d195. https://doi.org/10.1136/bmj.d195.

68. Mannion R, Davies H. Understanding organisational culture for healthcare quality improvement. *BMJ* 2018; 363: k4907. https://doi.org/10.1136/bmj.k4907.

69. Mannion R, Davies HTO, Marshall MN. Cultural characteristics of 'high' and 'low' performing hospitals. *J Health Organ Manage* 2005; 19: 431–39. https://doi.org/10.1108/14777260510629689.

70. Bate P. *Strategies for Cultural Change*. Oxford: Butterworth-Heinemann; 1994. https://doi.org/10.1016/C2013-0-04535-5.

71. West M, Dawson J, Admasachew L, Topakas, A. *NHS Staff Management and Health Service Quality: Results from the NHS Staff Survey and Related Data*. London: Department of Health; 2011. www.gov.uk/government/publications/nhs-staff-management-and-health-service-quality (accessed 30 March 2022).

72. Dixon-Woods M, Baker R, Charles K, et al. Culture and behaviour in the English National Health Service: overview of lessons from a large multi-method study. *BMJ Qual Saf* 2014; 23: 106–15. http://dx.doi.org/10.1136/bmjqs-2013-001947.

73. Curry LA, Brault MA, Linnander EL, et al. Influencing organisational culture to improve hospital performance in care of patients with acute myocardial infarction: a mixed-methods intervention study. *BMJ Qual Saf* 2018; 27: 207–17. http://dx.doi.org/10.1136/bmjqs-2017-006989.

74. Mannion R, Braithwaite J. Unintended consequences of performance measurement in healthcare: 20 salutary lessons from the English National Health Service. *Intern Med J* 2012; 42: 569–74. https://doi.org/10.1111/j.1445-5994.2012.02766.x.

Cambridge Elements ⧉

Improving Quality and Safety in Healthcare

Editors-in-Chief

Mary Dixon-Woods

THIS Institute (The Healthcare Improvement Studies Institute)

Mary is Director of THIS Institute and is the Health Foundation Professor of Healthcare Improvement Studies in the Department of Public Health and Primary Care at the University of Cambridge. Mary leads a programme of research focused on healthcare improvement, healthcare ethics, and methodological innovation in studying healthcare.

Graham Martin

THIS Institute (The Healthcare Improvement Studies Institute)

Graham is Director of Research at THIS Institute, leading applied research programmes and contributing to the institute's strategy and development. His research interests are in the organisation and delivery of healthcare, and particularly the role of professionals, managers, and patients and the public in efforts at organisational change.

Executive Editor

Katrina Brown

THIS Institute (The Healthcare Improvement Studies Institute)

Katrina is Communications Manager at THIS Institute, providing editorial expertise to maximise the impact of THIS Institute's research findings. She managed the project to produce the series.

Editorial Team

Sonja Marjanovic

RAND Europe

Sonja is Director of RAND Europe's healthcare innovation, industry, and policy research. Her work provides decision-makers with evidence and insights to support innovation and improvement in healthcare systems, and to support the translation of innovation into societal benefits for healthcare services and population health.

Tom Ling

RAND Europe

Tom is Head of Evaluation at RAND Europe and President of the European Evaluation Society, leading evaluations and applied research focused on the key challenges facing health services. His current health portfolio includes evaluations of the innovation landscape, quality improvement, communities of practice, patient flow, and service transformation.

Ellen Perry

THIS Institute (The Healthcare Improvement Studies Institute)

Ellen supported the production of the series during 2020–21.

About the Series

The past decade has seen enormous growth in both activity and research on improvement in healthcare. This series offers a comprehensive and authoritative set of overviews of the different improvement approaches available, exploring the thinking behind them, examining evidence for each approach, and identifying areas of debate.

Cambridge Elements ⁼

Improving Quality and Safety in Healthcare

Elements in the Series

Collaboration-Based Approaches
Graham Martin and Mary Dixon-Woods

Co-Producing and Co-Designing
Glenn Robert, Louise Locock, Oli Williams, Jocelyn Cornwell, Sara Donetto, and Joanna Goodrich

The Positive Deviance Approach
Ruth Baxter and Rebecca Lawton

Implementation Science
Paul Wilson and Roman Kislov

Making Culture Change Happen
Russell Mannion

Operational Research Approaches
Martin Utley, Sonya Crowe, and Christina Pagel

A full series listing is available at: www.cambridge.org/IQ

Printed in the United States
by Baker & Taylor Publisher Services